OVEREATING SELF-HELP BOOKS

HOLISTIC APPROACHES TO OVERCOMING OVEREATING

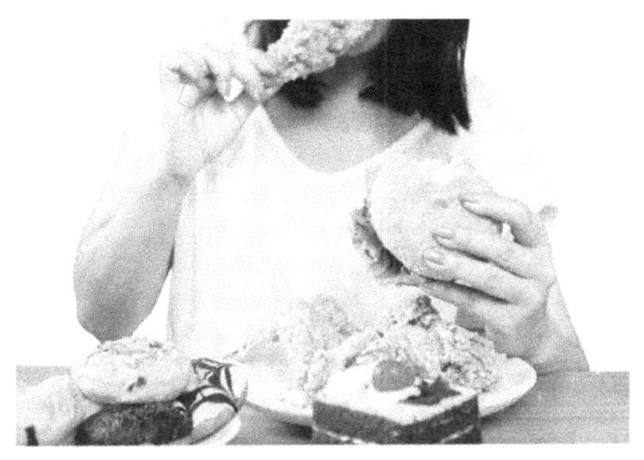

Author by
MIKE J CLACK

OVEREATING SELF HELP BOOKS

HOLISTIC APPROACHES TO OVERCOMING OVEREATING

Click on this link to view more and access books or scan the code thanks

https://www.amazon.com/author/mikeclackintlpublishe
r

TABLE OF CONTENTS

The paradox of excessive self-help because knowledge is readily available these days, the self-help sector has grown to be a multimillion-dollar business. Books in shops and online sellers proclaim to change every aspect of our lives, from our relationships and health to our jobs and economies. These books provide direction, motivation, and hope for a better, more satisfying life. But what happens if the need to improve oneself gets out of hand? When does the abundance of advice become more confusing than helpful? The following is the self-help overload paradox: This same contradiction is discussed in

"Overeating Self-Help Books: Holistic Approaches to Overcoming Overeating." While self-help books may be helpful resources for personal development, relying too much on them might result in a never-ending quest with little practical application. This is not simply another self-help book; rather, it offers advice on how to approach self-help books, especially those aimed at those who struggle with overeating, thoughtfully and in moderation. Recognizing the appeal of self-help literature

Why do we find self-help books so appealing? Everyone has a natural drive to improve and find answers to the problems they face in life. Self-help books provide practical actions that seem to be fast remedies, motivational tales, and organized guidance. They give us hope that by simply flipping the page, we can transform our lives and give us a sense of control in an otherwise chaotic environment.

THE PARADOX OF EATING TOO MUCH FOOD

The irony is that reading self-help books too much might have unexpected effects. Rather than

PART I: A JOURNEY TOWARDS BALANCE

This book aims to promote a more thoughtful and balanced approach, not to dissuade you from seeking self-help. You can maximize the effectiveness of self-help books by emphasizing quality over quantity and applying the principles you learn to your everyday life.

This path is about reaching a comprehensive sense of well-being that includes mind, body, and spirit, not simply about beating overeating. You'll find as you read these pages that the solutions you seek exist within you, not in the next book. We will investigate together how to realize your full potential and bring about enduring, constructive change.

Greetings from a fresh perspective on self-help. Greetings from the road to conquering overindulgence in food and finding equilibrium in an advice-filled environment.

OVERCONSUMPTION'S IRONY

It's easy to get into the overconsumption trap while pursuing self-improvement, especially when it comes to self-help literature. The irony of this overindulgence lies in the fact that while these books are supposed to help us improve, reading them too much might have the opposite impact.

Confusing instead of clarifying. We find ourselves paralyzed while acting. Seeking self-improvement via a never-ending supply of guidance often leaves us feeling more overwhelmed and less equipped to really make changes.

The Deception of Excellence, is the prospect of increased productivity and advancement is one of the primary reasons individuals pick up self-help books.

Every new book appears to contain the key to unlocking our potential, providing us with new perspectives and doable actions to help us accomplish our objectives. But reading book after book might give the impression that you are productive. Even if we are not doing anything to put what we have learned into practice, we may feel as if we are progressing just by taking in knowledge.

This variety has advantages and disadvantages. On the one hand, it provides a variety of viewpoints. However, it may result in contradictory recommendations. While some books encourage self-compassion and flexibility, others may advocate for rigorous discipline and set routines. Because of confusion and hesitation, readers are often left confused about which direction to choose as a consequence of confusion and hesitation.

We sometimes feel overwhelmed by the amount of information available to us, even with so many possible answers at our fingertips. We fail to take any significant action because we spend so much time examining and contrasting various tactics. This paralysis may be very harmful when it comes to problems like overeating, when prompt and definite action is essential for bringing about significant changes.

THE NEVER-ENDING CYCLE OF HUNTING

Overconsumption may also lead to procrastination, which is ironic. We don't put the advice from one book into practice; instead, we go on to the next, never quite finding the ideal answer. This never-ending search cycle may keep us from moving forward in a meaningful way. We become lifelong learners, never really acting but constantly practicing.

Ending the Cycle

It is crucial that we shift our attention from quantity to quality in order to escape the vicious cycle of overconsumption. Instead of reading every book there is, we may choose a handful that really speak to us and make a commitment to following their teachings. This entails approaching self-help with more mindfulness, reflecting on what we've read, and applying it to our lives.

Use in practice

By providing helpful tips for conscious reading and application, seeks to assist readers in resolving this conundrum. Through a comprehensive approach, this book addresses the underlying reasons for overeating and offers doable solutions that may be incorporated into everyday life. The intention is to promote a sensible and successful strategy rather than discourage reading self-help books.

Achieving Real Progress

In the end, the quality of our interactions with self-help books is what really matters, not how many of them we read. We may interrupt the pattern of excessive consumption and make real progress by emphasizing deliberate application as opposed to unending consumption. With so much advice available to us, this book is meant to support you along the way as you search for harmony, understanding, and long-lasting transformation.

As you set out on this journey, keep in mind that the solutions you seek may be found in how you choose to use the information you already have, not in the next book you pick up. Allow this book to walk by you as you shift from overindulgence to deliberate action, fostering a better connection between you and food.

HOW CAN YOU FIND BALANCE WITH THIS BOOK?

- It may be intimidating to navigate the self-help world, particularly if you feel like you're drowning in a sea of techniques, promises of change, and guidance.

- Holistic Approaches to Overcoming Overeating" is to steer you toward significant and long-lasting transformation while assisting you in finding equilibrium in the middle of this turbulence.

Finding the Inherent Reasons for Overeating

The complicated problem of overeating is impacted by mental, bodily, and spiritual aspects impact the complicated problem of overeating. This book takes a holistic approach to understanding and treating these underlying issues.

Emotional Triggers

Learn how your feelings affect the way you eat and how to deal with stress, anxiety, and other emotional triggers.

Physical Imbalances

Recognize the physiological effects of overeating, such as malnourishment, hormone imbalances, and other physical conditions that may influence your eating habits. Examine the concept of spiritual hunger and how overeating may result from a lack of spiritual satisfaction. Discover how to take care of your soul and discover a greater sense of fulfillment and significance in life.

Useful, implementable techniques

This book focuses on doable actions and techniques to make sure you can put what you learn into practice.

Mindful Eating Practices: Get tips on how to eat mindfully to improve your relationship with food. This entails eating with purpose, enjoying every meal, and being aware of hunger signs.

Goal Setting and Implementation: Learn how to make practical strategies to achieve your objectives and how to establish reasonable, attainable goals. This entails monitoring your progress and changing your strategy as needed.

Daily Schedules and Customs: Introduce fresh, healthy routines into your everyday routine. The book offers advice on how to establish habits that promote your general wellbeing and aid in avoiding overindulging in food.

Developing self-acceptance and compassion

Having a sympathetic connection with oneself is one of the keys to overcoming overeating. This book offers you guidance on developing acceptance and self-compassion.

Develop the ability to be kind and understanding to oneself, particularly while facing difficulties or disappointments. Give up on perfectionism and embrace self-forgiveness.

Make an effort to create a good self-image and a sound sense of value for yourself. Recognize the influence your self-perception has on your eating patterns and general health.

Including holistic methods

"Overeating Self-Help Books" highlights the importance of a comprehensive strategy that integrates the mind, body, and spirit in order to overcome overeating.

Examine the connections between your feelings, ideas, and bodily experiences. Use this knowledge to create plans that take care of every aspect of your well-being.

You may want to think about including mindfulness exercises, yoga, and meditation into your daily routine. These activities may help you achieve balance and reduce stress.

Promoting Conscientious Use of Self-Help Resources

This book also teaches you to use self-help resources more thoughtfully.

- Discover how to choose self-help books that really address your needs and objectives. Steer clear of the temptation of reading just for pleasure.
- Promote reflective practice by giving the advice you hear enough thought and by putting it into practice.

Prioritize the quality of your self-help journey above the quantity.

Bringing About Durable Change

The ultimate goal of this book is to help you bring about long-term change by applying its teachings and techniques to your daily life.

Rather than concentrating on band-aid solutions, make sustainable lifestyle changes. Recognize that sustained transformation requires effort and patience.

See personal growth as a lifelong process. Continue to develop, learn, and adjust as you go.

Your Journey Forward

This book aims to guide you toward a healthier relationship with food and a more balanced, fulfilling life. Let this book be the bridge between knowledge and action, helping you transform your understanding into meaningful and lasting change.

EMOTIONAL COMPONENT

In the world of weight management and healthy living, dieting has become synonymous with restriction, deprivation, and often, failure. Many people find themselves trapped in an endless cycle of dieting, losing weight, and then regaining it, often with a sense of frustration and defeat. This chapter is about breaking free from that cycle and embracing a healthy, sustainable relationship with food.

UNDERSTANDING THE DIETING TRAP

Dieting typically involves strict rules and limitations on what you can eat, often leading to short-term weight loss. However, this approach can have several negative consequences:

- **Yo-Yo Dieting:** The cycle of losing and regaining weight, known as yo-yo dieting, can be harmful to both physical and mental health. It can slow down your metabolism and increase the risk of developing eating disorders.

- **Nutritional Deficiencies:** Restrictive diets often eliminate entire food groups, leading to nutritional deficiencies that can impact overall health and well-being.

- **Emotional Toll:** Constantly monitoring food intake and adhering to strict rules can create a negative emotional relationship with food, resulting in guilt, anxiety, and stress around eating.

Shifting Your Mindset

To develop a healthier relationship with food, it's essential to shift your mindset from dieting to nourishment.

- **Focus on Nourishment:** Instead of thinking about what you can't eat, focus on what you can eat that will nourish your body. Choose foods that are rich in nutrients and that you enjoy.

- **Listen to Your Body:** Pay attention to your body's hunger and fullness cues. Eat when you are hungry and stop when you are satisfied, rather than following external rules.

- **Enjoy Food:** Allow yourself to enjoy food without guilt. Eating should be a pleasurable experience, not a source of stress.

PRACTICAL STRATEGIES FOR EMBRACING A HEALTHY RELATIONSHIP WITH FOOD

- Practice mindful eating by paying full attention to the eating experience. This means eating slowly, savoring each bite, and being aware of the flavors, textures, and aromas of your food.

- Aim for balanced meals that include a variety of nutrients. Incorporate plenty of vegetables, fruits, whole grains, lean proteins, and healthy fats into your diet.

- Stop labeling foods as "good" or "bad." All foods can fit into a healthy diet in moderation. Instead, focus on overall dietary patterns and making nutritious choices most of the time.

- Recognize when you are eating for emotional reasons rather than physical hunger. Develop alternative coping mechanisms for stress, boredom, or other emotions, such as exercise, hobbies, or talking to a friend.

- Develop positive rituals around food, such as cooking meals from scratch, enjoying meals with family or friends, and taking time to appreciate the food you eat.

LONG-TERM BENEFITS

By ditching dieting and embracing a healthy relationship with food, you can enjoy several long-term benefits:

Sustainable Weight Management without the pressure of dieting, you can achieve and maintain a healthy weight in a more natural and sustainable way.

A positive relationship with food can reduce stress and anxiety, improving overall mental health and well-being.

Better Physical Health and nourishing your body with a variety of nutrients can lead to better physical health, including improved energy levels, enhanced immune function, and reduced risk of chronic diseases.

Greater Enjoyment of Life, when food is no longer a source of stress or guilt, you can enjoy life more fully. Eating becomes a joyful, satisfying experience rather than a battleground.

PART II: CRACKING THE CODE OF EMOTIONAL EATING

Emotional eating is a common challenge that many people face. It involves using food to cope with feelings rather than to satisfy physical hunger. This behavior can lead to unhealthy eating patterns, weight gain, and a complicated relationship with food. Understanding and addressing emotional eating is crucial for developing a healthier relationship with food and achieving lasting well-being.

Emotional eating is often driven by the need to fill an emotional void or to distract from uncomfortable feelings. Common triggers include stress, boredom, sadness, loneliness, and even happiness. The act of eating can provide temporary comfort or distraction, but it doesn't address the underlying emotional issues.

- **Trigger:** An emotional trigger, such as stress or sadness, initiates the desire to eat.

- **Craving:** This trigger leads to a craving for specific foods, often those high in sugar, fat, or salt.

- **Eating:** Eating the desired food provides temporary relief or distraction from the emotion.

- **Aftermath:** After eating, feelings of guilt, shame, or regret may follow, often exacerbating the original emotional issue.

Identifying Emotional Triggers

The first step in overcoming emotional eating is to identify your specific emotional triggers. Keep a food diary to track what you eat, when you eat, and what emotions you experience before and after eating. Look for patterns and note any recurring themes.

- Work pressure, financial worries, and personal relationships can all contribute to stress-induced eating.

- Eating can become a way to pass the time when you feel bored or unoccupied.

- Emotional distress, such as sadness or depression, can lead to comfort eating.

- Eating can serve as a substitute for social interaction and companionship.

- Positive emotions, such as happiness and excitement, can also lead to overeating, especially during celebrations and social gatherings.

STRATEGIES TO OVERCOME EMOTIONAL EATING

- Physical activity is a great way to relieve stress and improve your mood. Find an activity you enjoy, such as walking, yoga, or dancing.

- Practice relaxation techniques like deep breathing, meditation, or progressive muscle relaxation to manage stress.

- Engage in hobbies that bring you joy and satisfaction, such as reading, painting, gardening, or playing a musical instrument.
- Reach out to friends, family, or support groups for connection and emotional support.

Mindful Eating Practices

Pause and Reflect before eating, pause and ask yourself if you are truly hungry or if you are eating in response to an emotion. Rate your hunger on a scale from 1 to 10.

Focus on eating mindfully by paying attention to the taste, texture, and aroma of your food. Eat slowly and savor each bite.

Serve yourself a reasonable portion and avoid eating directly from the package.

Healthy Emotional Expression

Write down your thoughts and feelings to gain insight into your emotional state and identify patterns.

Use creative outlets like art, music, or writing to express your emotions constructively.

Sometimes, talking about your feelings with a trusted friend or therapist can help you process and manage emotions without turning to food.

Structured Eating Patterns

Regular Meals eat regular meals and snacks to maintain stable blood sugar levels and reduce the temptation to eat emotionally.

Balanced Nutrition ensure your diet includes a balance of nutrients to keep your body satisfied and reduce cravings.

Building a Healthier Relationship with Food

By addressing the emotional triggers of overeating and developing healthier coping mechanisms, you can build a more positive relationship with food.

Practice self-compassion and be kind to yourself. Recognize that emotional eating is a common challenge and that it's okay to seek help and support.

Acknowledge and celebrate your progress, no matter how small. Each step towards healthier eating habits is a victory.

IDENTIFYING EMOTIONAL TRIGGERS AND PATTERNS

One of the critical steps in overcoming emotional eating is identifying the specific triggers and patterns that lead to this behavior. Understanding what drives you to eat emotionally can help you develop healthier strategies for coping with your emotions. This chapter will guide you through the process of identifying your emotional triggers and recognizing the patterns that contribute to emotional eating.

KEEPING A FOOD AND EMOTION DIARY

A highly effective tool for identifying emotional triggers and patterns is a food and emotion diary. This diary will help you track not only what you eat but also how you feel before and after eating.

1. Record Your Meals and Snacks: Write down everything you eat and drink, including portion sizes and meal times.

2. Note Your Emotions: Pay attention to your emotional state before and after eating. Were you feeling stressed, bored, lonely, happy, or sad? Record these emotions in your diary.

3. Identify Context and Situations: Include details about the context of your eating. Were you alone or

with others? Were you at home, at work, or somewhere else? What were you doing before you decided to eat?

4. Reflect on Physical Hunger: Rate your level of physical hunger on a scale from 1 to 10 before eating. This can help distinguish between physical hunger and emotional hunger.

Analyzing Your Diary

After keeping your diary for a week or two, review your entries to identify patterns and triggers. Look for recurring themes and situations that lead to emotional eating.

1. What Emotions Are Most Common? Are there specific emotions that frequently trigger your eating? For example, do you often eat when you're stressed, bored, or lonely?

2. What Times of Day Are Problematic? Do you notice a pattern in the times of day when you're more likely to eat emotionally? Perhaps late at night or during the mid-afternoon slump?

3. What Situations or Events Trigger Emotional Eating? Are there particular situations or events that prompt you to eat emotionally, such as work stress, family conflicts, or social gatherings?

4. What Types of Foods Do You Crave? Are there specific types of foods you crave when eating emotionally? For example, do you reach for sweets, salty snacks, or comfort foods?

Recognizing Emotional Eating Patterns

Understanding your emotional eating patterns involves recognizing the connections between your emotions, triggers, and eating behaviors.

- Stress Eating: You find yourself reaching for food when you feel overwhelmed by work, deadlines, or personal responsibilities. Stress often leads to cravings for high-fat, high-sugar foods that provide temporary comfort.

- Boredom Eating: You eat to fill the time when you're bored or have nothing else to do. This often happens in the evenings or on weekends when you have unstructured time.

- Comfort Eating: You use food as a way to soothe negative emotions such as sadness, loneliness, or anxiety. Comfort foods are typically those that remind you of happier times or provide a sense of security.

- Social Eating: You eat more than usual in social situations, either to fit in with others or because the presence of food is tempting. This can happen at parties, gatherings, or even casual get-togethers with friends.

- Celebratory Eating: You overeat during celebrations or when you're feeling particularly happy or excited. This pattern is often seen during holidays, birthdays, or special occasions.

STRATEGIES FOR MANAGING EMOTIONAL TRIGGERS

Once you've identified your emotional triggers and patterns, you can develop strategies to manage them without turning to food

1. Develop Healthy Coping Mechanisms: Replace emotional eating with healthier coping mechanisms. For example, if you eat when stressed, try stress-relief techniques like exercise, meditation, or deep breathing.
2. Plan for Trigger Situations: Prepare for situations that you know will trigger emotional eating. If social gatherings are a trigger, plan to eat a healthy

meal beforehand or bring nutritious snacks with you.

3. Create a Support System: Surround yourself with supportive people who can help you stay on track. Talk to friends, family, or a therapist about your emotional eating struggles.

4. Practice Mindfulness: Mindfulness can help you stay present and aware of your emotions without immediately reacting to them with food. Practice mindfulness techniques such as mindful breathing, body scans, or mindful eating.

5. Address Underlying Emotional Issues: Sometimes, emotional eating is a symptom of deeper emotional issues. Consider seeking professional help to address underlying problems such as depression, anxiety, or unresolved trauma.

THE PHYSICAL ASPECT
WHEN OVEREATING IS DRIVEN BY BODY IMBALANCE

Overeating can sometimes be driven by underlying imbalances within the body, including hormonal fluctuations, nutritional deficiencies, and other physiological factors. Understanding these imbalances is essential for addressing overeating and promoting overall well-being. This chapter explores common body imbalances that can contribute to overeating and offers strategies for restoring balance to the body.

Hormonal Imbalances

Hormones are essential for controlling energy balance, metabolism, and hunger.

Hormone imbalances, including insulin, cortisol, ghrelin, and leptin, may interfere with these functions and cause overeating. One hormone that controls energy balance and indicates fullness is called leptin.

When the body stops responding to leptin's signals, it might develop leptin resistance, which increases appetite and causes overeating.

Ghrelin promotes appetite, hence its nickname, "hunger hormone." Overeating may be caused by an imbalance in ghrelin levels, which can lead to excessive appetite and desires.

Insulin is critical for glucose metabolism and energy control. Overeating, elevated desires, and unstable blood sugar levels may result from insulin dysregulation or resistance. Often referred to as the "stress hormone," cortisol regulates metabolism and hunger.

Prolonged stress may cause cortisol levels to become dysregulated, which can then lead to emotional eating and overeating.

NUTRITIONAL DEFICIENCIES

Nutritional deficiencies can also contribute to overeating by disrupting the body's hunger and satiety signals. When the body lacks essential nutrients, it may crave specific foods in an attempt to fulfill its nutritional needs.

- Protein is essential for satiety and muscle repair. A deficiency in protein can lead to increased hunger and cravings for high-calorie foods.
- Fiber helps to promote feelings of fullness and regulate digestion. A lack of fiber in the diet can result in rapid spikes and drops in blood sugar levels, leading to increased hunger and overeating.

- Deficiencies in vitamins and minerals, such as vitamin D, vitamin B12, iron, and magnesium, can affect energy levels, mood, and appetite regulation, potentially leading to overeating.

STRATEGIES FOR RESTORING BALANCE

Addressing fundamental imbalances with dietary adjustments, targeted therapies, and lifestyle adjustments is necessary to bring the body back into balance.

Eat a diet high in whole, nutrient-dense foods, such as fruits, vegetables, whole grains, lean meats, and healthy fats, in a balanced manner. In order to promote general health and wellbeing, try to include a range of nutrients.

Eating well-balanced meals and snacks throughout the day can help you establish regular eating habits. This may lessen hyperbolic cravings and overindulgence in food while also stabilizing blood sugar levels.

Eat mindfully by taking your time, appreciating each meal, and being aware of your body's signals of hunger and fullness. Become attuned to your body's hunger and fullness signals instead of depending on outside stimuli.

Use relaxation methods to control your stress, such yoga, deep breathing, meditation, and time spent in nature. Make self-care activities that support emotional stability and relaxation a priority.

Exercise on a regular basis to promote metabolism and general wellness. Exercise may lessen cravings for unhealthy meals, elevate mood, and assist control hormones.

See a medical expert, such as a doctor or qualified dietitian, if you believe there may be underlying hormone imbalances or nutritional deficiencies. Based on your particular requirements, they may provide tailored treatments and suggestions.

UNDERSTANDING NUTRITIONAL NEEDS AND PHYSICAL HEALTH

Proper nutrition is essential for maintaining optimal physical health and well-being. Our bodies rely on a balanced diet rich in essential nutrients to support vital functions, such as energy production, metabolism, immune function, and tissue repair.

The Role of Nutrition in Physical Health

Nutrients like carbohydrates, fats, and proteins provide the energy needed for everyday activities, exercise, and metabolic processes.

Essential vitamins and minerals act as cofactors and antioxidants, supporting cellular function, DNA repair, and immune response.

Protein is crucial for building and repairing muscle tissue, supporting muscle growth, strength, and recovery.

Calcium, vitamin D, and other nutrients play a vital role in maintaining strong and healthy bones, reducing the risk of osteoporosis and fractures.

A balanced diet low in saturated fats and cholesterol and rich in fiber, antioxidants, and omega-3 fatty acids can help reduce the risk of heart disease and improve cardiovascular health.

Omega-3 fatty acids, antioxidants, and other nutrients support brain health, cognitive function, and mood regulation.

Essential Nutrients for Physical Health

To maintain optimal physical health, it's essential to consume a variety of nutrients from different food sources.

- Protein is essential for building and repairing tissues, supporting muscle growth, and maintaining a healthy immune system.
- Carbohydrates are the body's primary source of energy and provide fuel for physical activity and brain function.
- Healthy fats, such as omega-3 fatty acids and monounsaturated fats, are important for brain health, hormone production, and the absorption of fat-soluble vitamins.
- Vitamins are essential micronutrients that play a variety of roles in the body, including immune function, energy metabolism, and antioxidant defense.

- Minerals are essential for various physiological functions, including bone health, muscle contraction, nerve transmission, and fluid balance.
- Fiber is crucial for digestive health, regulating bowel movements, maintaining healthy cholesterol levels, and promoting satiety.

Dietary Recommendations for Optimal Health

To meet your nutritional needs and promote overall physical health, follow these dietary recommendations

- Consume a diverse range of nutrient-rich foods, including fruits, vegetables, whole grains, lean proteins, and healthy fats.
- Include a balance of carbohydrates, proteins, and fats in your diet, focusing on high-quality sources of each nutrient.

- Minimize consumption of processed and ultra-processed foods high in added sugars, unhealthy fats, and sodium.

- Drink plenty of water throughout the day to stay hydrated and support proper bodily functions.

- Pay attention to portion sizes and avoid oversized servings to prevent overeating and promote weight management.

- Tune into your body's hunger and satiety cues, eating when hungry and stopping when satisfied.

STRATEGIES FOR PROMOTING OVERALL WELLNESS

- Engage in regular exercise and physical activity to support cardiovascular health, muscle strength, flexibility, and mental well-being.

- Prioritize quality sleep to support physical recovery, hormone regulation, immune function, and cognitive performance.

- Practice stress-reduction techniques such as meditation, deep breathing, yoga, or spending time in nature to support overall well-being.

- Cultivate meaningful relationships and social connections to promote emotional health, reduce stress, and increase feelings of happiness and fulfillment.

- Schedule regular check-ups with your healthcare provider for preventive screenings, vaccinations, and health assessments.

- If you suspect underlying hormonal imbalances or nutritional deficiencies, consider seeking guidance from a healthcare professional, such as a doctor, registered dietitian, or naturopathic physician. They can assess your individual needs, perform diagnostic tests if necessary, and provide personalized recommendations and interventions to restore balance to your body.

- Explore holistic approaches to restoring balance to the body, such as acupuncture, herbal medicine, massage therapy, or chiropractic care. These complementary therapies can help address imbalances in the body's energy systems, promote relaxation, and support overall well-being.

- Incorporate self-care practices into your daily routine to nurture your physical, mental, and emotional well-being. This may include activities like journaling, spending time in nature, practicing gratitude, engaging in creative pursuits, or taking regular breaks to rest and recharge.

- Restoring balance to the body is a gradual process that requires patience and persistence. Be consistent with implementing healthy habits and give yourself grace along the way. Celebrate small victories, listen to your body's feedback, and trust in your ability to support your overall health and well-being.

THE SPIRITUAL DIMENSION

In addition to physical and emotional needs, humans also have spiritual needs that are essential for overall well-being and fulfillment. Recognizing spiritual hunger involves acknowledging a deeper longing for meaning, purpose, connection, and transcendence. This chapter explores the concept of spiritual hunger, its significance in our lives, and strategies for addressing it to achieve greater spiritual fulfillment.

Understanding Spiritual Hunger

Spiritual hunger is the longing for something beyond the material realm, a desire for connection to something greater than oneself. It manifests as a deep inner yearning for meaning, purpose, belonging, and transcendence. While spiritual hunger is often associated with religious beliefs and practices, it can also be experienced in a secular context as a quest for existential meaning and fulfillment.

Signs of Spiritual Hunger

- A sense of emptiness or inner void despite external accomplishments or possessions.
- A deep desire to understand the purpose and meaning of life, existence, and one's place in the universe.
- A yearning for deeper connections with oneself, others, nature, or a higher power.
- Questioning beliefs, values, and assumptions about the nature of reality, existence, and the divine.
- Craving experiences of awe, wonder, and transcendence that evoke a sense of connection to something greater than oneself.
- Wrestling with existential questions about life, death, suffering, and the nature of reality.

STRATEGIES FOR ADDRESSING SPIRITUAL HUNGER

Allocate time for introspection and self-examination to delve into your core wants, values, and beliefs. You may develop a connection with your inner knowledge and intuition via journaling, meditation, or silent reflection.

To strengthen your spiritual connection with the natural world, spend time outside. Get outside and do something awe-inspiring, like hiking, gardening, or just sitting in quiet.

Develop present-moment awareness and strengthen your spiritual connection by incorporating mindfulness activities into your everyday routine.

Engaging in body scans, mindful walking, and mindful breathing may facilitate your connection to the sanctity of every moment. Investigate using creative expression to establish a connection with your deepest emotions, ideas, and spiritual encounters.

Take up artistic pursuits to convey your innermost desires and dreams, such as writing, painting, dancing, or music. Seek out connections and groups that encourage your spiritual development and provide chances for growth, connection, and joint inquiry. Attend retreats, conversation groups, and spiritual events to meet others who share your beliefs.

Develop a feeling of empathy and connectivity by engaging in acts of service and compassion. Take part in charity donations, volunteer labor, or deeds of kindness to improve the lives of others and promote spiritual contentment.

Investigate holy writings, lessons, and wisdom traditions that align with your spiritual principles and convictions.

Read books on philosophy or religion, go to seminars or lectures, and converse with spiritual mentors or instructors.

Take part in contemplative activities to strengthen your spiritual connection and cultivate a feeling of respect and devotion, such as meditation, prayer, chanting, or rituals.

Fulfilling the Soul: Going Beyond Food Food feeds the body, but feeding the soul, heart, and intellect nourishes the spirit, which consists of the deeper aspects of our existence.

Spiritual Sustaining Taking care of one's spiritual needs and fostering a feeling of interconnectedness with something bigger than oneself are essential components of spiritual sustenance. It includes activities and encounters that awaken the soul, inspire amazement and wonder, and promote a greater comprehension of life's mysteries.

Techniques for Providing Spiritual Support

Take up meditation and other reflective exercises to calm your thoughts, develop inner tranquility, and establish a connection with your deepest self. Investigate various meditation techniques, such as guided visualization, loving-kindness meditation, and mindfulness meditation.

Accept ritual, prayer, and holy rites as means of recognizing life's sanctity and establishing a connection with the divine. Create devotional activities, candle lightings, or prayer recitations as part of your own routines that speak to your values and beliefs.

To strengthen your connection with nature and invigorate your soul, spend time outside. To appreciate the grandeur and beauty of creation, go on walks in the forest, relax by the sea, or look up at the stars at night. Investigate artistic expression as a way to establish a connection with your deepest emotions, ideas, and spiritual encounters.

Take up creative pursuits such as writing, painting, dancing, or music to communicate your innermost desires. Develop a feeling of empathy and connectivity by engaging in acts of service and compassion. Engage in community service, show compassion to others, or donate to worthy charities to improve people's lives and promote spiritual contentment.

Investigate philosophical viewpoints, teachings, and wisdom traditions that align with your values and spiritual convictions. To learn more about the deeper secrets of life, study holy literature, go to seminars or lectures, and have discussions with spiritual mentors or instructors.

Adopt a mindful lifestyle to infuse daily tasks with awareness and presence. Develop an awareness of the present moment in your relationships, household tasks, and recreational pursuits by practicing mindfulness.

CULTIVATING MEANING AND PURPOSE

By engaging in practices that nourish the spirit, we cultivate a deeper sense of meaning, purpose, and fulfillment in life. We awaken to the interconnectedness of all beings, embrace life's mysteries with curiosity and wonder, and find solace in the beauty and richness of the human experience.

Practices for Spiritual Fulfillment

Spiritual fulfillment is cultivated through intentional practices that nourish the soul, deepen our connection to the divine, and awaken a sense of purpose and meaning in life. In this chapter, we explore a variety of practices that can support your journey towards spiritual fulfillment and inner peace.

Cultivate an attitude of gratitude by focusing on the blessings and abundance in your life. Start each day with a gratitude practice, reflecting on the things you are thankful for. Keep a gratitude journal to record your blessings and moments of grace, and notice how gratitude transforms your perspective and outlook on life.

Explore wisdom teachings and spiritual traditions that resonate with your soul's longing for truth and understanding. Dive into sacred texts, attend lectures or workshops, and seek out spiritual mentors or teachers who can guide you on your journey. Embrace the wisdom of the ages and allow it to illuminate your path.

Practice being fully present in each moment, cultivating awareness and acceptance of whatever arises. Let go of regrets about the past and worries about the future, and instead focus on the richness of the present moment. Cultivate presence in your relationships, your work, and your daily activities, allowing the fullness of life to unfold.

Making Peace with Food and Yourself

1. Cultivating Self-Compassion and Acceptance

Self-compassion and acceptance are essential practices for nurturing inner peace, resilience, and well-being. In this chapter, we explore the importance of treating ourselves with kindness and understanding, and we offer strategies for cultivating self-compassion and acceptance in our lives.

2. Understanding Self-Compassion

Self-compassion involves treating ourselves with the same kindness, care, and understanding that we would offer to a dear friend in times of struggle or suffering. It involves recognizing our own humanity, embracing our imperfections, and offering ourselves unconditional love and support.

3. Embracing Acceptance

Acceptance involves acknowledging and embracing all aspects of ourselves, including our strengths, weaknesses, successes, and failures. It involves letting go of self-judgment, comparison, and the need to be perfect, and instead, embracing ourselves exactly as we are in this moment.

STRATEGIES FOR CULTIVATING SELF-COMPASSION AND ACCEPTANCE

By bringing awareness to your thoughts, emotions, and sensations without passing judgment, you may cultivate self-compassion and mindfulness. Give yourself some love and support, and remember that you're doing the best you can and that it's OK to suffer.

Take up self-compassionate meditation techniques that emphasize developing compassion, warmth, and understanding for oneself. Breathe deeply and settle into the present moment while repeating loving affirmations like "May I be kind to myself" or "May I accept myself as I am".

Maintain a self-compassion notebook in which you record times when you have struggled or faced difficulties and address them with words and deeds that reflect self-compassion. Think back to instances in which you have been nice to yourself and accept your inherent value and deservingness.

Make self-care practices that feed your body, mind, and soul a priority. Take part in things that make you happy, calm, and refreshed; some examples of these are having a bath, taking a stroll in the park, or spending time with close friends and family.

Let go of the urge to be flawless and set reasonable standards for yourself. Acknowledge your limits, faults, and experiences as inevitable aspects of being human. Whatever the result, acknowledge and appreciate your efforts and growth.

By concentrating on the positive aspects of your life and yourself, you may cultivate an attitude of appreciation for your path and yourself. Write three things every day for which you are thankful, including traits about yourself that you find admirable, in a gratitude diary.

Seek assistance from loved ones, friends, or a therapist who can provide you with empathy, comprehension, and affirmation. Knowing that you're not alone and that help is on hand, be honest about your troubles and obstacles. Forgive yourself for the errors you've made in the past and any apparent shortfalls. Give yourself forgiveness and understanding for being a human instead of self-blame, guilt, and anger.

Changing the Way You Think About Food

There are many different facets to our connection with food, including cultural, social, emotional, and physiological influences. We discuss the significance of reframing our relationship with food in this chapter in order to advance wellbeing, happiness, and health.

We provide knowledge and methods for developing a more nutritional, balanced, and mindful eating style.

Recognizing Your Connection with Food

Consider your connection with food and take note of any patterns, attitudes, or actions that could be affecting the way you eat. Think about how your connection with food is shaped by your emotions, stress levels, body image, and previous food experiences.

Engage in mindful eating by appreciating the tastes, textures, and scents of your food as well as the whole sensory experience of eating. Chew your meal well, eat slowly, and pay attention to your body's signals of hunger and fullness. When dining, try not to get distracted by activities like watching TV or browsing through your phone. Instead, concentrate on the food at hand.

Accept intuitive eating as a means of reestablishing communication with your body's natural intelligence and hunger cues. Eating when you are physically hungry and stopping when you are comfortably full are ways to honor your appetite. Instead than depending on outside guidelines or limitations, trust your body to help you make nourishing and satisfying eating choices.

Giving Up Food Shame and Guilt

Embrace a loving and nonjudgmental mindset toward yourself and your eating habits to let go of guilt and shame related to food. Understand that food is not inherently "good" or "bad," and that a diversified and balanced diet may include a variety of foods. When you stray off course or make decisions that are at odds with your health objectives, remember to be kind to yourself and provide forgiveness.

Dismissing Diet Culture

Take issue with diet culture and the ubiquitous messaging that encourage restriction, weight reduction, and unattainable body goals. Prioritize self-care routines and health-promoting activities that enhance your general well-being above external measurements of value, such as beauty or weight.

Getting Satisfied and Enjoying Your Food

Give yourself permission to indulge in your favorite meals without feeling guilty or constrained, and rediscover the joy and fulfillment that comes with eating. Instead than focusing on strict guidelines or outside expectations, concentrate on the pleasure that comes with eating as an experience. Try different tastes, cooking methods, and cuisines to enhance the enjoyment and satisfaction of eating.

Looking for Assistance and Advice

If you're having trouble redefining your relationship with food, get help and advice. To build a better connection with food, think about collaborating with a licensed dietician, therapist, or counselor who can provide you with individualized techniques and resources. Accompanying yourself on your path with accountability and support might also come from joining a support group or community of like-minded people.

Give your food some thought and pause before you start eating. Take note of the food's hues, textures, and scents as it is presented to you. Give thanks for the food it offers and the work that went into making it.

As you eat, use every sense. Take note of each bite's warmth, texture, and flavor. Take note of the noises made while chewing and swallowing. Consider the arrangement of the food on your plate. You may improve your perception and pleasure of the food by devoting yourself entirely to the sensory experience.

Eat mindfully and slowly, in tiny bites. Savor every bite of food, giving careful consideration to its tastes and textures. By eating more slowly, you may improve your awareness of your body's signals of hunger and fullness, which can help you avoid overindulging and aid in digestion.

Throughout the meal, periodically check in with your body. Take note of any bodily feelings, such as contentment, fullness, or hunger. Observe how your body reacts to various meals and respect its cues by eating in accordance with your own requirements and preferences.

Eat with an attitude of **non-judgment**, devoid of guilt or condemnation. Give up on ideas and opinions about what constitutes "good" or "bad" food and concentrate instead on providing your body with nourishment from meals that promote your overall health and wellbeing. Remember to be kind and compassionate to yourself, and remember that moderation is the key to enjoying any meal.

Establish a calm and distraction-free dining space. Switch off all electronics, take a break from work or other activities, and focus only on eating. You may totally immerse yourself in the present and enjoy the feeling of fueling your body by limiting distractions.

Give thanks for the nutrition that comes from the meal you're consuming. Consider the path that food takes from the field to your plate, appreciating the work that farmers, producers, and chefs put into getting it to you. Developing an attitude of thankfulness may improve your dining experience and strengthen your connection with the food you consume.

Pay attention to your body's signals of hunger and fullness; eat when you're really hungry and stop when you're satisfied. Pay attention to your body's signals of hunger and contentment rather than eating out of habit, boredom, or emotion. You may create a more harmonious and balanced relationship with food by listening to the knowledge of your body.

FREEING YOURSELF FROM THE PAST

Addressing Past Trauma and Its Impact on Eating Habits

Past trauma can have a profound impact on our relationship with food and eating habits, often leading to disordered eating patterns, emotional eating, or other forms of maladaptive coping mechanisms. In this chapter, we explore the connection between past trauma and eating behaviors and offer strategies for healing and fostering a healthier relationship with food.

Understanding the Impact of Trauma

Trauma can take many forms, including physical, emotional, or sexual abuse, neglect, accidents, natural disasters, or witnessing violence. These experiences can leave lasting psychological and emotional wounds that impact various aspects of our lives, including our relationship with food and our bodies.

Recognizing Trauma-Related Eating Behaviors

1. Emotional Eating: Using food as a way to cope with difficult emotions or numb painful feelings.
2. Restrictive Eating: Restricting food intake as a means of exerting control in response to feelings of powerlessness or vulnerability.
3. Binge Eating: Consuming large quantities of food in a short period, often as a way to soothe emotional distress or fill a void.

4. Avoidance of Food: Avoiding certain foods or food-related situations due to trauma-related triggers or associations.

5. Body Dissatisfaction: Developing negative body image or disordered eating patterns as a result of trauma-related shame or self-esteem issues.

Healing from Trauma and Nourishing Self-Compassion

You may want to think about getting help from a trauma expert, therapist, or counselor who can provide you with healing techniques, affirmation, and direction.

Therapy can help you learn healthier coping techniques, recognize dysfunctional coping strategies, and process traumatic events. As you go through the healing process, practice kindness and self-compassion.

Realize that the way you eat is an adaptive way for you to cope with the trauma in your past, and that you deserve compassion and encouragement as you recover.

Learn to be mindfully aware of your thoughts, feelings, and eating habits without passing judgment or criticizing yourself. Examine other methods of dealing with discomfort, and take note of any patterns or triggers that lead to eating habits connected to trauma.

See food not as a source of guilt or punishment, but as a means of self-care and nutrition. In order to relish and appreciate the flavors and textures of your food, practice mindful eating and concentrate on eating balanced meals that feed your body and mind.

As you go through the healing process, surround yourself with kind and understanding people who can validate, encourage, and empathize with you. Look for local trauma survivors' support groups so you can meet others who have gone through similar things.

Try using artistic, musical, literary, or movement mediums to communicate and work through your trauma-related feelings.

Self-expression, empowerment, and healing are some of the benefits of artistic expression. Acquire and use grounding methods, such as progressive muscle relaxation, deep breathing, or meditation, to help stabilize your nervous system and treat symptoms resulting from trauma.

Grounding exercises may help you feel more in control of your emotions, more focused, and more present.

Methods for Letting Go and Moving on Moving on from the past and into the future is a powerful process that helps us let go of emotional burdens, end destructive habits, and welcome a better future.

1. Put acceptance into action. Acceptance is the first step in letting go and moving forward. Recognize the truth of your prior experiences, along with whatever suffering or letdown you may have had. Recognize that accepting yourself as you are does not involve endorsing or justifying prior experiences; rather, it only acknowledges them as a part of your narrative.

2. Work on forgiveness. Being able to forgive releases us from the burden of grudges, rage, and bitterness. It is a transforming discipline. Give yourself and others the benefit of the doubt about any perceived wrongs or injuries. Recall that forgiving yourself frees you from the weight of holding grudges and

enables you to go on with an open heart. Forgiveness is a gift that you offer yourself.

3. Let go of attachments. Releasing ties to people, circumstances, or results that no longer benefit us is often necessary in order to let go. Determine the expectations or attachments you may have been holding onto, then practice letting them go with kindness and love. Have faith that letting go of attachments makes room for fresh starts and personal development.

4. Engage in mindfulness exercises. By focusing attention on the here and now, mindfulness is an effective technique for letting go and moving on. To ground oneself in the present moment, engage in body scan methods, deep breathing exercises, or mindfulness meditation. You may develop a feeling of serenity and clarity that helps you let go of the past by keeping your attention on the present.

5. Establish limits. Setting limits gives us the ability to safeguard our mental health and satisfy our needs, which is a crucial part of letting go and moving on. Determine which relationships or circumstances are draining your energy or compromising your morals, then set firm boundaries to protect your boundaries and encourage positive connections.

6. Accept yourself with compassion. Letting go of self-criticism and adopting a more loving and caring connection with oneself requires self-compassion. Try being kind and patient with yourself; treat yourself with the same love and understanding you would show a close friend going through a similar situation. Remind yourself that you deserve to be loved and accepted for who you are.

7. Practice self-care. Taking care of yourself is crucial if you want to support your body, mind, and soul throughout the process of letting go and moving on. Make it a priority to make time for the things that

make you happy, calm, and refreshed. These might include yoga, nature walks, hobbies, and spending time with close friends and family. By taking care of yourself, you can restock your inner reserves and develop resilience in the face of hardship.

8. Pay attention to possibility and growth. Change your focus from moping over the past to looking forward to what lies ahead. Create a growth mindset that sees obstacles as opportunities for knowledge acquisition and development. Establish objectives that will spur you on, and take aggressive measures to fulfill your goals and desires. By concentrating on development and possibilities, you can build up good momentum that moves you forward on your journey.

BUILDING A RESILIENT AND POSITIVE SELF-IMAGE

Our well-being is based on having a resilient and positive self-image, which gives us the ability to face life's obstacles with grace, certainty, and confidence.

Self-compassion is the foundation of a resilient and positive self-image. Especially in tough or self-doubting moments, be kind, understanding, and accepting of yourself.

Accept your flaws and errors as necessary components of your path, and treat yourself with the same kindness you would a close friend. Recognize when you are talking negatively to yourself, and gently and impartially address it. When you catch yourself being judgmental or critical of yourself, replace those negative ideas with words that are encouraging and reassuring.

Develop a more realistic and balanced self-perception that acknowledges both your areas of success and your need for progress in addition to your abilities, skills, and qualities. Recognize and appreciate your abilities, successes, and skills.

Recognize your special talents and attributes, and be proud of the person you are growing into.

Develop an attitude of gratitude and self-appreciation for the traits and abilities that make you unique.

Establish attainable objectives that are consistent with your beliefs, passions, and dreams.

Divide more ambitious objectives into more doable segments, and acknowledge and appreciate your accomplishments as you go. You may boost your self-efficacy, confidence, and sense of competence by creating and completing important objectives.

Resilience is the ability to overcome hardship and grow stronger as a result. Develop your resilience by recognizing obstacles and failures as opportunities for improvement.

Adopt a development attitude that views setbacks and failures as transient roadblocks to achievement.

Focusing on the benefits and richness of your life can help you cultivate an attitude of appreciation.

Every day, set aside some time to consider your blessings, whether they be important events, enduring relationships, or individual successes.

Having gratitude in your life helps you change your perspective from what's missing to what's plentiful and present.

Be in the company of people who inspire and uplift you, such as mentors, encouraging friends, and role models. Look for settings and pursuits that promote happiness, contentment, and optimism.

Minimize your exposure to harmful influences, such as unwholesome relationships or demeaning media. Make self-care routines that feed your body, mind, and soul a priority.

Take part in joyful, restorative, and rejuvenating activities; these might include physical activity, meditation, artistic endeavors, or time spent in nature. You can boost your resistance to life's obstacles and replenish your vitality by taking care of yourself.

Setting Realistic and Achievable Goals

- Define Your Vision
- Clarify Your Objectives
- Visualize Success
- Break it Down
- Divide into Milestones

(Your Goal Should Be SMART)

- Set Deadlines

- Measurable

- Achievable

- Relevant

- Time-bound

- Stay Flexible

- Be Open to Adjustments

- Celebrate Progress

- Seek Support

- Enlist Support

- Find an accountability Partner

Implementing Sustainable Lifestyle Changes

Identify Your Priorities: Determine what areas of your life you want to change or improve.

Focus on Incremental Progress: Begin with small, manageable changes to build momentum and confidence.

Gradually Increase Difficulty: As you become comfortable with new habits, challenge yourself to take on more ambitious goals.

Prioritize Long-Term Sustainability: Select lifestyle changes that are practical, enjoyable, and compatible with your daily routine.

Consider Environmental Impact: Opt for practices that minimize waste, conserve resources, and promote environmental sustainability.

Nourish Your Body: Focus on consuming nutritious foods, staying hydrated, getting regular exercise, and prioritizing sleep.

Practice Mindfulness: Incorporate mindfulness techniques such as meditation, deep breathing, or journaling to reduce stress and enhance well-being.

Enlist Supportive Allies: Surround yourself with friends, family, or online communities who share similar goals and can offer encouragement and accountability.

Seek Professional Guidance: Consult with healthcare professionals, nutritionists, or certified coaches for personalized advice and support.

Monitor Your Results: Keep track of your progress using journals, apps, or other tracking tools to stay motivated and accountable.

Celebrate Milestones: Acknowledge and celebrate your achievements along the way to maintain motivation and momentum.

MAINTAINING MOTIVATION AND OVERCOMING SETBACKS

Change your viewpoint and see failures as important teaching moments that will make you stronger and smarter.

When things are tough, treat yourself with the same love and understanding that you would if a friend were going through a difficult period.

Speak with mentors, family members, or friends who may provide support, direction, and a sympathetic ear.

Make connections with others who share your aims and experiences by using social media, online forums, or support groups.

By taking a step back and modifying your tactics appropriately, evaluate what's working and what isn't.

Recognize that growth may not always be linear and remain adaptable. Give oneself room to develop and learn from failures.

Make sure you are surrounded by inspirational materials, such as books, podcasts, inspirational quotations, or tales of people who have succeeded in overcoming comparable obstacles.

Imagine the person you want to be, and let that image motivate you to keep moving ahead in the face of challenges.

UNDERSTANDING INTERNAL CONFLICTS AND SELF-SABOTAGE

Recognize when your goals or desires are in conflict with each other, causing inner turmoil and indecision.

Dig deeper to understand the underlying beliefs, fears, or past experiences that contribute to internal conflicts.

Become aware of patterns of behavior that undermine your goals or lead to self-destructive outcomes.

Confront self-sabotaging thoughts and behaviors with compassion and objectivity, seeking healthier alternatives.

Treat yourself with kindness and understanding, offering yourself the same empathy you would give to a friend facing challenges.

Let go of guilt or shame associated with past mistakes, recognizing that they are opportunities for growth and learning.

Learn healthy ways to cope with stress, triggers, and setbacks without resorting to self-sabotaging behaviors.

Embrace setbacks as opportunities for growth and resilience, bouncing back stronger and wiser from challenges.

Seek support from friends, family, or professionals who can offer guidance, encouragement, and perspective.

Connect with others who are facing similar challenges, sharing experiences and strategies for overcoming self-sabotage.

BUILDING INNER STRENGTH AND RESILIENCE

- Recognize Patterns
- Explore Triggers

Common Self-Sabotaging Behaviors

Procrastination: Putting off tasks or responsibilities, leading to missed opportunities or increased stress.

Negative Self-Talk: Engaging in self-criticism, doubt, or pessimism, eroding confidence and motivation.

Avoidance: Dodging challenges or uncomfortable situations, preventing growth and progress.

Perfectionism: Setting impossibly high standards, leading to frustration, burnout, or paralysis.

Self-Isolation: Withdrawing from social connections or support networks, increasing feelings of loneliness and disconnection.

Escapist Behaviors: Using substances, distractions, or unhealthy coping mechanisms to numb emotions or avoid reality.

Recognizing Warning Signs

- Notice signs of stress, anxiety, or tension in your body, such as headaches, muscle tension, or digestive issues.
- Pay attention to feelings of guilt, shame, or self-doubt that accompany self-sabotaging behaviors.
- Observe changes in behavior, such as increased irritability, impulsivity, or mood swings.

- Share your struggles with trusted friends, family members, or professionals who can offer support and guidance.

- Connect with others who are dealing with similar challenges, sharing experiences and strategies for overcoming self-sabotage.

Identifying Self-Sabotaging Behaviors

- Become aware of behaviors that undermine your goals or lead to self-destructive outcomes.

- Identify situations, emotions, or beliefs that trigger self-sabotage, such as fear of failure or low self-esteem.

- Setting impossibly high standards, leading to frustration, burnout, or paralysis.

- Withdrawing from social connections or support networks, increasing feelings of loneliness and disconnection.

- Using substances, distractions, or unhealthy coping mechanisms to numb emotions or avoid reality.

CREATING A SUPPORTIVE ENVIRONMENT FOR SUCCESS

Spend time with people who encourage and inspire you. Positive relationships can provide motivation, support, and valuable feedback.

Reduce time spent with individuals who are critical, unsupportive, or bring you down. This helps maintain a positive mindset and focus on your goals.

Establish a Conducive Physical Space

Keep your workspace and living areas tidy and organized. A clutter-free environment can improve focus and productivity.

Surround yourself with items that inspire you, such as motivational quotes, vision boards, or meaningful objects.

Develop a Routine

Establish a daily routine that includes time for work, rest, and self-care. Consistency can help build momentum and reduce stress.

Incorporate activities that nurture your physical, mental, and emotional well-being, such as exercise, meditation, or hobbies.

Seek Out Resources and Opportunities

Engage in continuous learning and development. Take courses, attend workshops, or read books related to your goals.

Utilize tools and resources that can help you achieve your goals, such as apps, online communities, or professional services.

Set Clear Goals and Monitor Progress

Set clear, specific, and achievable goals. Having a clear direction can increase motivation and focus.

Regularly review and assess your progress towards your goals. Adjust your strategies as needed to stay on track.

Encourage Accountability

Partner with someone who can help keep you accountable to your goals. Regular check-ins can provide motivation and support.

The Power of Present-Moment Awareness

Present-moment awareness, also known as mindfulness, involves focusing your attention on the here and now, fully engaging with the current experience without judgment.

This practice helps reduce stress, enhance emotional regulation, and improve overall well-being by preventing the mind from dwelling on the past or worrying about the future.

Benefits of Being Present

Reduced Stress by focusing on the present moment, you can alleviate anxiety and stress that often stem from future uncertainties or past regrets.

Present-moment awareness sharpens your concentration and enhances your ability to perform tasks more effectively.

Being present allows you to experience emotions fully and respond to them appropriately, leading to better emotional health.

Engaging fully with your current experiences increases your appreciation and enjoyment of everyday moments.

Focus on your breath, observing each inhale and exhale without trying to change it. This can anchor your mind in the present.

Pay attention to different parts of your body, starting from your toes and moving up to your head, noticing any sensations without judgment.

Choose an object in your environment and observe it closely, noticing its details, colors, and textures as if seeing it for the first time.

Listen to the sounds around you without labeling them or getting caught up in thoughts about them. Simply experience the act of listening.

Integrating Mindfulness into Daily Life

Savor each bite of your meal, paying attention to the flavors, textures, and sensations. This can enhance your enjoyment of food and promote healthier eating habits.

Pay attention to the sensations in your body as you walk, the feeling of your feet touching the ground, and the sights and sounds around you.

Engage fully in conversations, listening attentively and responding thoughtfully without getting distracted by your own thoughts or judgments.

Overcoming Challenges in Mindfulness Practice

Developing present-moment awareness takes time and practice. Be patient with yourself and persist even if it feels challenging initially.

Approach your mindfulness practice with a non-judgmental attitude. Accept whatever thoughts and feelings arise without criticism.

Mindful Breathing

Sit comfortably, close your eyes, and take slow, deep breaths. Focus your attention on the sensation of your breath entering and leaving your body. When your mind wanders, gently bring it back to your breathing.

Inhale through your nose for 4 seconds, hold your breath for 7 seconds, and exhale through your mouth for 8 seconds. Repeat this cycle several times to center yourself.

Body Scan Meditation

Lie down comfortably and focus on each part of your body, starting from your toes and moving up to your head. Notice any sensations, tension, or relaxation in each area.

Spend a few minutes paying attention to your entire body as a whole, noticing how it feels in the present moment without trying to change anything.

Mindful Observation

Select an everyday object, such as a flower or a cup. Observe it closely, noticing its color, shape, texture, and any other details. Engage with the object as if you are seeing it for the first time.

Take a walk outside and pay close attention to your surroundings. Notice the colors of the leaves, the sound of birds, and the feeling of the ground beneath your feet.

Mindful Listening

Choose a piece of music or listen to the sounds around you. Focus entirely on the listening experience, noticing the different layers of sound and any emotions or thoughts that arise.

Sit quietly and listen to the ambient sounds around you. Allow yourself to hear each sound fully, without labeling or judging it.

Mindful Eating

Eat a meal or snack slowly, savoring each bite. Notice the taste, texture, and smell of the food. Pay attention to the act of eating without distractions such as TV or smartphones.

Before eating, take a moment to appreciate the food in front of you. Reflect on the journey it took to reach your plate and the nourishment it provides.

Mindful Movement

Practice yoga with a focus on the breath and body alignment. Move slowly and mindfully through each pose, paying attention to how your body feels.

Walk slowly and deliberately, paying attention to the sensations of each step. Notice how your feet feel as they make contact with the ground and how your body moves.

Mindful Communication

When conversing with someone, give them your full attention. Listen without planning your response or interrupting. Notice the speaker's words, tone, and body language.

Speak slowly and clearly, choosing your words mindfully. Be aware of the impact your words have on others and strive to communicate with kindness and clarity.

Daily Mindfulness Practices

Spend a few minutes each day writing about your thoughts, feelings, and experiences. Reflect on your entries to gain insights into your mindfulness journey.

At the end of each day, take a few minutes to reflect on your experiences. Consider moments when you felt present and mindful, and think about how you can cultivate more of these moments.

Incorporate mindfulness into daily routines, such as brushing your teeth or washing dishes. Focus on the sensations and actions involved in these tasks.

Begin your day by setting a mindful intention. This could be a simple goal, such as "I will be present during my meetings today" or "I will take deep breaths when I feel stressed."

Incorporating Mindfulness into Daily Life

Begin your day with a short meditation session. Spend 5-10 minutes focusing on your breath and setting a positive intention for the day.

Practice positive affirmations each morning. Repeat statements like "I am calm and focused" or "I will approach today with mindfulness and presence."

Eat slowly and mindfully. Pay attention to the taste, texture, and aroma of your food. Chew thoroughly and appreciate each bite.

Take a moment before eating to express gratitude for your meal. Reflect on the effort that went into growing, preparing, and serving the food.

Incorporate yoga or stretching into your daily routine. Focus on your breath and the sensations in your body as you move through each pose.

Practice walking meditation, either indoors or outdoors. Walk slowly and mindfully, paying attention to each step and the contact of your feet with the ground.

Take short breaks throughout the day to practice deep breathing. Inhale deeply through your nose, hold for a few seconds, and exhale slowly through your mouth.

Whenever you feel stressed or distracted, take a moment to focus on your breath. Observe the natural rhythm of your breathing without trying to change it.

PART IV: HOLISTIC APPROACHES

Mind-Body Techniques

Regular meditation helps reduce stress, improve concentration, and enhance overall well-being. Practice mindfulness meditation, guided visualization, or loving-kindness meditation.

Yoga combines physical postures, breath control, and meditation to promote physical and mental health. Different styles, such as Hatha, Vinyasa, or Yin yoga, can be tailored to individual needs.

This ancient Chinese martial art focuses on slow, deliberate movements and deep breathing. Tai Chi enhances balance, flexibility, and mental clarity.

Energy Healing

Reiki: A Japanese technique for stress reduction and relaxation that also promotes healing. Practitioners use their hands to transfer healing energy to the patient, balancing their energy fields.

Acupuncture: A traditional Chinese medicine practice that involves inserting thin needles into specific points on the body to balance the body's energy, or Qi, and alleviate various ailments.

Qi Gong is a holistic system of coordinated body posture, movement, breathing, and meditation used for health, spirituality, and martial arts training.

Nutritional Therapy

Consuming a diet rich in whole, unprocessed foods like fruits, vegetables, whole grains, and lean proteins supports overall health and vitality.

Herbal Medicine: Using plants and plant extracts to treat and prevent illnesses. Herbal remedies can support various aspects of health, from boosting the immune system to reducing inflammation.

Functional Nutrition: Tailoring dietary plans based on individual health needs, considering how diet, environment, and lifestyle factors influence health and wellness.

Emotional and Spiritual Healing

Writing down thoughts, feelings, and experiences helps process emotions, gain insights, and promote mental clarity and emotional well-being.

Aromatherapy: Using essential oils extracted from plants to promote physical and emotional health. Oils can be inhaled, applied to the skin, or used in baths to enhance mood and well-being.

Engaging in spiritual practices such as prayer, meditation, or attending religious services can provide comfort, purpose, and a sense of community.

Physical Therapies

Massage Therapy: Manipulating the body's muscles and soft tissues to relieve pain, reduce stress, and promote relaxation and healing.

Chiropractic Care: Adjusting the spine and other parts of the body to correct alignment issues, relieve pain, and support the body's natural ability to heal.

Hydrotherapy: Using water in various forms (steam, ice, liquid) for pain relief and treatment of illness.

Practices include hot baths, saunas, and cold compresses.

Lifestyle Practices

Engaging in regular physical activity, such as walking, swimming, or strength training, improves physical health, mood, and energy levels.

Ensuring sufficient, quality sleep is crucial for overall health. Practice good sleep hygiene, such as maintaining a regular sleep schedule and creating a restful environment.

Incorporating mindfulness into daily activities, such as eating, walking, and working, enhances awareness, reduces stress, and improves quality of life.

Integrating Mind-Body-Spirit Techniques

Practice mindfulness meditation daily to cultivate present-moment awareness and reduce stress. Focus on your breath, observe your thoughts without judgment, and gently bring your attention back to the present whenever it wanders.

Use positive affirmations to reinforce self-belief and promote a positive mindset. Repeat statements like "I am strong and capable" or "I embrace the present moment" each day.

Spend a few minutes each day visualizing your goals and desired outcomes. Imagine yourself achieving these goals and experiencing the associated positive emotions.

Body Techniques

Incorporate yoga into your routine to connect mind and body. Yoga postures (ASANAS), breath control (pranayama), and meditation (DHYANA) help improve flexibility, strength, and mental clarity.

Practice Tai Chi regularly to enhance physical balance, coordination, and mental focus. The slow, deliberate movements promote relaxation and a sense of inner peace.

Spirit Techniques

Dedicate time to spiritual meditation or prayer. Focus on connecting with a higher power or your inner self to gain insight, peace, and spiritual nourishment.

Spend time in nature to nourish your spirit. Activities like hiking, gardening, or simply sitting in a park can help you feel grounded and connected to the earth.

Cultivate gratitude by keeping a gratitude journal. Each day, write down three things you are thankful for, which can enhance your spiritual well-being and foster a positive outlook on life.

Understanding Alternative Therapies

Alternative therapies encompass a variety of treatment approaches that fall outside conventional Western medicine. They focus on holistic healing and often emphasize the connection between mind, body, and spirit.

These therapies can complement traditional medical treatments, offering benefits such as reduced stress, improved mental health, enhanced physical well-being, and overall balance.

Common Alternative Therapies

- *Acupuncture* involves inserting thin needles into specific points on the body to balance energy flow (Qi). It is used to treat various conditions, including pain, stress, and digestive issues.

Benefits can alleviate chronic pain, reduce migraines, improve sleep, and enhance overall well-being.

- ***Chiropractic care*** focuses on diagnosing and treating musculoskeletal disorders, particularly spine misalignments, through manual adjustments. The benefit Can relieve back and neck pain, improve posture, enhance joint mobility, and promote overall health.

- Uses plant-based remedies to treat and prevent illnesses. Herbs can be consumed as teas, capsules, extracts, or applied topically. It Supports immune function, reduces inflammation, and addresses specific health concerns naturally.

- A form of energy healing where practitioners use their hands to transfer healing energy to the recipient, balancing their energy fields.

Promotes relaxation, reduces stress and anxiety, and enhances overall emotional and physical well-being.

- *Aromatherapy* Uses essential oils extracted from plants for therapeutic purposes. Oils can be inhaled, applied to the skin, or used in baths.

Can improve mood, alleviate stress, enhance sleep quality, and support respiratory health.

- **Homeopathy** Based on the principle of "like cures like," homeopathy uses highly diluted substances to trigger the body's natural healing response.

It Addresses chronic conditions, supports immune function, and offers a gentle approach to healing with minimal side effects.

- *Massage Therapy* Involves manipulating the body's muscles and soft tissues to relieve pain, reduce stress, and promote relaxation and healing.

Alleviates muscle tension, improves circulation, enhances lymphatic drainage, and promotes mental relaxation.

- ***Naturopathy*** Emphasizes natural remedies and the body's self-healing ability. Naturopathy includes diet and lifestyle changes, herbal medicine, and other holistic approaches.

Treats the root cause of illnesses, supports long-term health, and promotes a holistic approach to wellness.

Integrating Alternative Therapies

1. Consult Professionals and Ensure that practitioners of alternative therapies are certified and experienced in their fields. Consult with your healthcare provider before starting any new therapy.

Personalized Plans with professionals to create personalized treatment plans that address your specific health needs and goals.

Combine with Conventional Medicine

Use alternative therapies alongside conventional treatments for a comprehensive approach to health. Inform your healthcare providers about all therapies you are using.

Regularly assess the effectiveness of the therapies and make adjustments as needed to ensure optimal results.

Educate Yourself Learn about different alternative therapies, their benefits, and potential risks. Read books, attend workshops, and consult reliable sources to make informed decisions.

Incorporate self-care practices such as mindfulness, yoga, and nutrition to support your overall health and enhance the effectiveness of alternative therapies.

Finding What Works for You

Begin by assessing your physical, emotional, and spiritual health. Identify specific issues or areas you want to improve, such as chronic pain, stress, or overall well-being.

Clearly define your health and wellness goals. Whether you aim to reduce anxiety, improve sleep, or enhance your overall vitality, having clear objectives will guide your exploration of alternative therapies.

Educate yourself about various alternative therapies, including their benefits and potential risks. Resources such as books, reputable websites, and educational videos can provide valuable information.

Look for case studies, testimonials, and reviews from individuals who have tried different therapies. Personal experiences can offer insights into the effectiveness and practicality of each therapy.

Consulting Professionals Consult with healthcare providers, holistic health practitioners, or therapists who specialize in alternative treatments. They can offer professional guidance tailored to your specific health needs.

Consider working with an integrative health practitioner who combines conventional medicine with alternative therapies. This holistic approach ensures that all aspects of your health are addressed.

DEVELOPING HEALTHY ROUTINES AND HABITS

Routines provide structure and stability, helping you manage your time effectively and reduce stress.

Consistent habits lead to sustained health benefits, whether it's improved physical health, mental clarity, or emotional well-being.

Identify what you want to achieve with your routines, such as better sleep, increased energy, or reduced stress.

Divide your goals into manageable steps. For example, if you want to improve fitness, start with a daily 10-minute walk.

CREATING A BALANCED ROUTINE

Morning Routine

Wake Up Early: Aim to wake up at the same time each day to regulate your body's internal clock.

Hydrate: Start your day by drinking a glass of water to kick start your metabolism and rehydrate after sleep.

Nutrition and Hydration

Balanced Meals: Eat a balanced diet rich in fruits, vegetables, whole grains, lean proteins, and healthy fats. Plan your meals ahead to ensure you get the necessary nutrients.

Regular Meals: Eat at regular intervals to maintain energy levels and avoid overeating. Don't skip breakfast, as it provides the energy you need to start your day. Drink plenty of water throughout the day.

Aim for at least 8 glasses, adjusting based on your activity level and climate.

Evening Routine

Create a relaxing evening routine to signal your body that it's time to sleep. This could include reading, taking a warm bath, or practicing gentle yoga.

Reduce exposure to screens at least an hour before bed to improve sleep quality. The blue light from devices can disrupt your sleep patterns.

Aim for 7-9 hours of sleep each night. Go to bed and wake up at the same time every day, even on weekends.

Developing Positive Habits

Begin with small, manageable changes. Gradual adjustments are more sustainable and less overwhelming.

Practice new habits consistently. It takes time for a habit to become automatic, typically around 21 days.

Keep a journal or use a habit-tracking app to monitor your progress and stay motivated.

Overcoming Challenges

Recognize potential barriers to developing healthy routines and find ways to overcome them. For example, prepare meals in advance if time is a constraint.

Be adaptable. Life is unpredictable, so it's important to adjust your routines when necessary without feeling discouraged.

Share your goals with friends or family members who can offer encouragement and accountability.

Maintaining Motivation

Acknowledge and celebrate your progress, no matter how small. This positive reinforcement helps maintain motivation.

Use visual cues, such as sticky notes or reminders on your phone, to keep you focused on your goals.

Treat yourself when you reach milestones. Rewards can be small, like enjoying a favorite activity or a healthy treat.

Continuous Improvement

Periodically reflect on your routines and habits. Assess what's working and what needs adjustment to better align with your goals.

Continuously educate yourself about health and wellness to stay inspired and informed about best practices.

Make self-care a non-negotiable part of your routine. Prioritize activities that nourish your mind, body, and spirit.

BALANCING WORK, REST, AND PLAY

Balancing work, rest, and play is essential for holistic well-being. It ensures you stay productive, relaxed, and fulfilled.

Maintaining balance helps prevent burnout, reduces stress, and promotes long-term health and happiness.

Work: Maximizing Productivity

Prioritize Task, Identify and prioritize your most important tasks each day. Use tools like to-do lists or task management apps to stay organized.

Break Tasks into Steps and Divide larger tasks into smaller, manageable steps to make them less overwhelming and more achievable.

Time Management Allocate specific blocks of time for different tasks. This helps you stay focused and ensures that important tasks get completed.

Avoid Multitasking and Focus on one task at a time to improve efficiency and the quality of your work.

Taking Breaks

Use the Pomodoro Technique—work for 25 minutes, then take a 5-minute break. After four cycles, take a longer break. This improves concentration and productivity.

Take regular breaks to stretch, walk, or do something enjoyable. This helps refresh your mind and body, enhancing overall productivity.

THE IMPORTANCE OF COMMUNITY AND CONNECTION

Building Support Systems

Communities provide comfort and a feeling of belonging, both in good and difficult times. It may promote resilience and lessen stress, depending on one's support network.

Developing interactions with other individuals promotes mental health and happiness by fending off feelings of isolation and loneliness.

Promoting growth and expansion. Through the interchange of ideas, experiences, and information, communities provide chances for education, development, and personal advancement. Communities that collaborate encourage innovation, creativity, and idea sharing, all of which promote development and advancement in all directions. encouraging the health of the body and the mind. Fostering relationships and participating in community events may improve physical health by promoting active, healthy lifestyles and convenient access to resources and assistance.

Emotional intelligence and a feeling of belonging are associated with improved mental health outcomes, including lower rates of stress, anxiety, and depression. Creating a welcoming atmosphere Social groups provide environments in which individuals, regardless of their appearance, background, or viewpoint, are respected, included, and welcomed. As members of a community, people may help each other discover their identity and purpose and maybe contribute to something greater than themselves.

Developing Partnerships Strong friendships, life-improving experiences, and cherished memories are fostered by communities. Additionally, they support people in developing meaningful relationships. When support, guidance, and help are needed, those with close community links may depend on one another to provide them. strengthening the community. Social cohesion and stability are achieved by communities fostering collaboration, mutual respect, and trust between disparate groups of people. Engaging with the public sphere

A deeper sense of community and constructive social change are fostered by volunteerism, civic engagement, and advocacy, all of which are more prevalent in vibrant communities. Overcoming obstacles Communities provide a structure for collective resilience, which makes it possible for people to band together and help one another during difficult times like crises or natural disasters.

Resolving issues: Communities may successfully handle local difficulties and find solutions to complicated issues by combining their resources, skills, and experience. Developing empathy and compassion Assisting people in discovering and connecting to their varied viewpoints and life experiences, belonging to a community helps individuals develop empathy and compassion for others. Social peace and general well-being are improved when communities foster compassion and kindness through deeds of charity, solidarity, and unity. Giving the place a feeling. By establishing and creating regional identities, customs, and cultures, local identity promotes a sense of pride and belonging in a specific location.

The general experience of the group is enhanced by public spaces like parks and libraries, which act as centers of celebration, interaction, and teamwork.

YOUR JOURNEY FORWARD

Understand that real well-being involves more than simply physical health. Aim for harmony and balance in your spiritual, emotional, and mental lives. In order to support total well-being, holistic wellness integrates a variety of lifestyle aspects, such as relationships, interactions with others, relationships with food, exercise, stress management, and personal growth.

Recognize that your path to holistic wellbeing is unique and very personal. As you make your way toward health, embrace your uniqueness and respect your needs, preferences, and beliefs. Along the journey, cultivate self-acceptance and self-compassion.

Treat yourself with respect, acknowledge your accomplishments, and draw compassionate, understanding lessons from your setbacks. Practice mindfulness by giving your experiences your full attention and being in the present. Stress is lessened, self-awareness is increased, and a closer connection with both the outside world and oneself is fostered by practicing mindfulness.

Incorporate mindfulness into every element of your life, including your career, relationships, and diet and exercise routines. You may appreciate life's little moments, handle stress better, and make deliberate decisions that promote your wellbeing by leading a mindful life.

Make deep connections with others a priority, and foster relationships that are encouraging. Participate in groups that share your interests and beliefs, and surround yourself with positive and inspiring people.

Encourage a strong connection with the natural world. Spend time outside and in natural settings to experience the wonder and beauty of the earth's scenery. Make taking care of yourself a priority every day.

Take care of your physical, emotional, mental, and spiritual needs by engaging in activities like regular exercise, a good diet, mindfulness, art, and spiritual upkeep. Allocate time for pursuits that provide happiness, satisfaction, and a sense of direction. Take part in passion projects, artistic endeavors, and pastimes that uplift and feed your spirit.

Recognize that achieving holistic wellbeing involves a lifetime of personal development, evolution, and self-exploration. Remain devoted to your own development, accept and welcome change and metamorphosis, and have an open mind to fresh opportunities for recovery and progress.

Maintain your curiosity and keep studying about wellness, holistic health, and personal growth. Discover new viewpoints, methods, and therapies that speak to you, and then incorporate them into your quest for well-being. You may follow your intuition and inner knowledge to achieve holistic wellbeing.

Make decisions that are consistent with your core beliefs and values by paying attention to your body's cues and respecting your inner wisdom. Recall that you possess the ability to manifest the life and well-being you want.

Give yourself the tools you need to take charge of your health and wellbeing and have faith in your capacity to create a life that is vibrant, balanced, and fulfilling.

Greetings, Reader I want to sincerely thank you for joining me on my path towards holistic wellbeing by reading these pages. It is a delight to share with you ideas, methods, and approaches that may completely change the way you live, not simply your health.

Holistic health is an ongoing process of self-awareness, development, and empowerment rather than a static endpoint. It's about achieving harmony and balance in all areas of your life—not only your physical body but also your mind, heart, and soul.

You will discover a plethora of knowledge, motivation, and useful tools on these pages to help you along the way. Each chapter provides direction and inspiration to help you flourish in all aspects of your life, from embracing self-care and respecting your own path to developing mindfulness and creating meaningful relationships. Never forget that you are the creator of your own health narrative. With one decision and one action at a time, you possess the ability to design a life full of energy, pleasure, and fulfillment.

As you read these words, I encourage you to embrace the transforming possibilities that lie ahead, believe in your path, and pay attention to your inner knowledge.

I hope that this book will be a help and a guide for you as you pursue holistic wellbeing. I hope it motivates you to take care of your body, reawaken your soul, and live each day with intention, fervor, and awareness. With appreciation and best wishes for your travels,

Mike J. Clack

REQUEST FOR BOOK REVIEW

"Overeating Self Help Books: Holistic Approaches to Overcoming Overeating"

An evaluation of "Overeating Self-Help Books: Holistic Approaches to Overcoming Overeating" is underway. Respected Reviewer, Since I'm writing this,

I hope you're doing well. I, Mike J. Clack, am the author of the newly published book "Overeating Self-Help Books: Holistic Approaches to Overcoming Overeating." My purpose in reaching out to you is to request a review of my book. Within "Overeating Self-Help Books," I delve into the subtleties of binge eating and provide practical, comprehensive remedies. Having a balanced relationship with food, body, and self is made possible by the skills this book imparts to its readers.

It is the result of years of research and firsthand knowledge. A few of the subjects addressed in an attempt to promote a healthy and joyful life include emotional eating comprehension, physical imbalance treatment, and soul nutrition. Given your knowledge and ability in, I believe you would provide a perceptive assessment of my work. Your review would not only help potential readers understand the value and relevance of the book to their own lives, but it would also provide constructive feedback. I'd be glad to provide you with a free copy of the book if you'd rather have a hard copy than an electronic one. If you're interested, tell me about your preferred format and mailing address. If you have one, please let me know. Thank you for giving thought to my request. Although I really appreciate your time and thoughtfulness, I am looking forward to your evaluation. Respectfully, Clack, Michael J.